POWER
ISO-BOW
30 SECOND
Method

POWER ISO-BOW 30 SECOND

Method

The Best Isotonic/Isokenetic Exercises that build muscle mass, increase strength, and sculpt the best body Lifelong!

BECOME A ISO-BOW MAN!

The Power Iso-Bow 30 Second Method was written to help you get closer to your physical potential when it comes to real muscle sculpting strengthening exercises. The exercises and routines in this book are quite demanding, so consult your physician and have a physical exam taken prior to the start of this exercise program. Proceed with the suggested exercises and information at your own risk. The Publishers and author shall not be liable or responsible for any loss, injury, or damage allegedly arising from the information or suggestions in this book.

Power Iso-Bow 30 Second Method
muscle-building Course

By

Birch Tree Publishing
Published by Birch Tree Publishing

Power Iso-Bow 30 Second Method
Published in 2020, All rights reserved,
No part of this book may be reproduced, scanned,
or distributed in any printed or electronic form without permission.

Birch Tree Publishing

Dedication

For Popeye Spinach **STRENGTH**, the quest **CONTINUES!**

Contents

GET "ISO-BOW" STRONG

Introducing the worlds fastest health and physique enhancing system

Introduction by John Hughes

I have been involved with athletics all of my life, from college wrestling to World Championship Master's Wrestling in my 60s. Coupled with over 15 years of high school coaching, I have always strived for top physical performance in strength and flexibility for myself and the athletes I coached. I purchased my first Bullworker in the 1960s and was impressed with how quickly my body responded to Bullworker strength training. The portability of the product meant I never had to get rid of it due to space restraints and over the next 30 years, the ability to supplement any exercise routine with a quick Bullworker workout, always complimented my desired fitness goal.

In 1999, I became the North American distributor for Bullworker and began to work on design changes to make the product much more challenging, yet always maintaining the portability aspect of this time tested and proven fitness product. In recognizing the importance of cross-training principles for maximum fitness results, I designed additional products that kept with the Bullworker portability concept with each product able to be used either separately or combined for maximum fitness results in a complete cross-training program.

In 2010, I purchased most of the Global rights to Bullworker and have reintroduced Bullworker training principles that have been effective since 1962 and resulted in over 10 million units sold. Proven as the ultimate portable fitness products, Bullworker continues to deliver results to everyone, any age, wherever they exercise.

Today, I present the Iso-Bow. This book is about transforming your body, mind and spirit, which is what health, strength and physique enhancement is all about.
I am really excited and positive to say that once you try the programs in this book, you will make some of the best gains you've ever made.
Join the men and women that are already using The Bullworker Power Series and programs with great success. **GET TRANSFORMED** today.

Keep pulling and pushing

Yours in Strength and Power

John Hughes

The Iso-bow 30 Second Method triggers as much muscle stimulation as quickly as possible, with up-to-the-minute exercise plans. You will be amazed at how easy it is to add strength, firm those muscles, and get lean in the comfort of your own home. Plus, you will see and feel your muscles getting leaner and fuller while gaining strength and, it will not take hours per day to accomplish this. You will get very fit even if you have limited time to do it. How? My program shows a simple muscle-coaxing-tactic that will activate significantly more growth fibers and will build lean muscle much faster with effective isometric contractions with the Iso-Bow.

The 30 Second Method is a spectacular condensed exercise and information book that gets the muscle-sculpting job done. There are exercise plans and explanations on how muscles grow and the reason they create additional strength and size gains. This book covers muscle fiber enhancement, my muscle expansion method, and how to activate and coax the muscle pump.

You can absolutely change your body in just minutes a day. I've been helping hundreds of trainees just like you to get in shape since 1995, and I've learned what it takes to get the body of your dreams in the shortest time possible. Consistent effort along with a positive mental attitude–coupled with this well-thought-out muscle-building-exercise plan, is all you need to acquire your goal - even after your first workout!

I've been doing this for a long time. So, I am confident with the program within these pages. To be honest people over complicate things with getting fit, building stronger muscles, and losing body-fat. This is the take: There are tons of multi-million-dollar-fitness facilities in almost every town or city around the world. Personal training studios and boot-camp facilities are popping up everywhere. Even bodybuilding and weight-loss supplements are readily available at supermarkets these days.

Fitness and muscles have taken over the world, however obesity is still by far relevant today. As a Professional fitness trainer and bodybuilder, I stand by the fact that the fitness industry has a lot to do with this mess. Theres massive competition with the latest exercise machines, magic pills, and magic exercise systems to get the consumer smaller without actual work. People are not sure what to do or who to believe in what really works from what does not. People do not understand how to do things to get what they want. So, that's where I come in.

The 30 Second Method is exactly what you need to focus on. I will take you back when Charles Atlas was the only fitness authority everyone wanted to be and look like. I followed in his footsteps along with millions of young men and women. Charles Atlas was getting the world in shape with a simple protocol that included self resistance and calisthenics along with a great attitude!

I am not Charles Atlas, but my 30 Second Method will work for you because it's based on sound fundamental basics. It is by far the safest method for developing muscles, gaining strength and increasing power for a fit and healthy life.

Now, the first time I ever saw an Isometric contraction performed was in March 1991, I was 17 years old. I've been exercising long before that with Dynamic Tension exercises along with pullups and other movements. The occasion was meeting up with body-builder Glenn Anderson. Glenn showed several isometric exercises and was a massive believer of isometrics and decline pushups! So, being extremely motivated, I continued with the program Glenn showed me.

A few months later, I met a guy called St Louis, that gave me a book on The Bullworker. Of course, St Louis heard all my stories on Charles Atlas and Dynamic Tension exercises and laughed. However, St Louis thought I would enjoy this book and gave it to me, which straight away I memorized page by page and exercise by exercise. I gave the course a good run using my Dynamic Tension type exercises instead of the Bullworker and adjusted the isometric holds.

Soon after that, my Uncle Ian showed up at the family home. He would flex his biceps for me and say, "boy Lou, you are getting bigger boy"! Which was the best compliment my uncle ever gave me to be honest. So I showed my uncle what I was doing, and he stated, you will only get stronger not bigger. I paid no attention for I knew my progress was far greater than his words, so I kept exercising and made a bet with my uncle. Which I won months later.

Months flew by, and I gave all the Isometric exercises a good run. Soon my results spoke for themselves, I became one of the most perfectly sculpted muscled-boy you could imagine. Now all my uncles had exceptional physiques; however, only Uncle Ian lifted weights. To me they all looked like muscular bodybuilding statues. But it was my uncle Rufus that was far leaner than all the three brothers. One day I said "Boff (which was my uncle's nickname), what have you been doing to get muscles like that"?

"Marlon," said my uncle, "I do isometric exercises every day but more in the last little while, and you are not the only one that has noticed the change." Now, let me say, I saw the change and I've kept doing it ever since. Today in the palms of your hands contain the master-plan to what I've learned throughout the years, and how to build strength, power and muscle size with the Iso-bow.

Continuing with the story, my uncle then tensed his forearm muscles in a way that seemed surreal to me. At first, all I saw was veins and ripped cords of muscle. He said grab my arm and squeeze it. I then felt the layers of muscle tense from inner to outer like an inflated balloon being blown up. My uncle's forearm muscles were fully engaged; it felt like his forearm had turned to granite. Normally, when you squeeze someones' arm, even when they are tense, there is some softness to the outer layers of tissue.

Uncle Boff explained that he had developed a high level of control over his muscles. He said tense, so I did and he told me that when most people tense up, they use only a fraction of their muscle fibers. Boff also said that people's inability to control more of their muscle fibers limited their functionality and strength. Boff stated to develop true strength one need to master the tension at will inside the muscle.

The greater the force generation and control, the greater the strength increases you will receive. This Isometric/Isotonic book will teach you how to control your muscles, for we have so much more control than we realise.. This form of training will condition you from the inside out.

Meaning, you will control not only your muscles, but your emotions as well. Simple issues will not bother you any more. The more you practice, the more control you will gain in every aspect of your life. That is the foundation of the program. The key is to incorporate the principles of Isometric Power into your daily routine. You will gain greater control over your life and learn how to let things go that you really need to.

This element took awhile for me to develop, but when you do, it is the key to self mastery. I do not base this on controlling everything in your life. It is about controlling your reaction to various situations you face on a day-to-day basis, so you can procure and experience greater fulfillment and joy in your life. That's why this book was written.

Best in Strength and Power

Marlon Birch

Chapter 1:
DEVELOPING SELF MASTERY

How the Iso-bow develops power

Gain Popeye Strength levels with Iso-Bow

01 DEVELOPING SELF MASTERY

Isometric exercises trigger as much chiseled muscle growth and strength as possible in quick, no-time-wasted bursts. It is the fastest way of stimulating as much muscle growth as possible within a short space of time. How? With the new Iso-Bow 30 Second Method which proves that my "efficient workouts" can help you activate significantly more lean growth fibers—and build muscle much faster with effective Mini-Hyper-Growth phases.

You will use quick, effective 30 Second Method routines for every targeted muscle in your exercise program— each time. These Hyper-Growth workouts will allow optimal recovery time to keep you progressing threefold. The full Iso-bow 30 Second programs are spectacular at triggering serious strength gains with workouts that get the muscle-sculpting job done in double quick time.

For example, the new 30 Second Method is my favorite stress method in this muscle-sculpting-protocol. As most readers know, I've been doing Isometric exercises and self resistance lifelong. So when it comes to results and effective training programs, which will make you work each muscle from one or two specific positions to ensure optimum-muscle-activation. The Iso-bow Isotonic Power contractions are efficient as is.

However, I've made it even better and faster by reconfiguring stress tactics based on more experimentation and research. It's the perfect solution to a condensed program, making it even more efficient at coaxing and increasing lean sculpted ripped to the bone muscle mass.

Before out-lining various programs, I'd like to explain how your muscles will be coaxed and the programs in this book are based on—and the reason it creates lean powerful (muscle-growth). You will learn about myofibrillar thickening, sarcoplasmic expansion and muscle-coaxing-fiber activation, the keys to increasing optimum fiber stimulation.

01 DEVELOPING SELF MASTERY

My goal with this book is not to provide you with a reference book on isometric exercises. Nor is it to put you on some random schedule or regime to "triple your strength in 2 months". Instead, I am looking at reshaping the way you look at the world. I want you to see possibilities where you never saw them before. When you are finished with this book, you realize that you are not done with the information in this book.

Practice and consistency is the name of the game here for self mastery. Progress takes time; and each day of pleasant practice, you will automatically see a huge difference. You will, however, gain control over your muscles and increase your strength and physique tremendously. Daily you will feel and see the strength gains and physique changes, day by day and week by week.

This program is layed out in such a way that anyone can do it. It is simple, yet challenging to the musculature. The workouts will not take long at all. You can perform all the exercises, take a shower, and perhaps cook a meal and get on with your day. Faster than getting in your car, driving to the gym car-park working out and driving back home again.

One More Thing: How much strength to apply: When performing these isotonic and isometric contractions, make sure you start out slow. Contract the muscles by pulling and pushing with light to medium tension for the desired effect. As you progress, you may start pulling and pushing slightly harder but please not too hard. Stimulate the muscles, do not annihilate them!

How Should You Read This book? I recommend reading this book in its entirety before starting the exercise routines. There are some key elements that could be detrimental to your practice and your connective tissues if not done correctly. For example, holding your breath while doing isometrics could make you pass out. Plus raise your blood pressure. The 30 Second Method is about mastering your muscle strength through your contraction.

01 DEVELOPING SELF MASTERY

What is Isometrics? Isometrics are exercises where your joints do not move. Normally with isotonic exercises, you move your joints through a full or partial range of motion. Think of the pullup, for example. You start off hanging from a bar and slowly raise yourself until your chin is above the bar. With isometric exercises, you stay in a fixed position.

Isotonics and Isometrics Increase Muscle Size: How can you gain more density and strength with the Iso-bow 30 Second protocol? First you will gain strength because my program emphasize on development of the myofibrils, the force-generating strands in muscle fibers. Then density because of increased force under load, by holding the contraction longer to increase the tension time on muscle and connective tissues.

The focus is on expanding the sarcoplasm, the energy fluid inside muscle fibers where glycogen, ATP and the mitochondria is housed. Enhancing density and strength are important elements to maximize muscle size and strength. The dominant fiber type in all of us is the fast-twitch-endurance-type 2As. They contain dual-capacity fibers with both endurance and strength components to increase muscle size. We have been brainwashed into thinking lifting weights and using a low rep range is the only way for us to get big muscles, not anymore. Today we have the Iso-Bow 30 Second Method.

There are loads of Isometric books on the market with 7 second contractions using excessive force to build muscles with isometrics. That's a fallacy and one of the main reasons muscle increases are very slow or most times non-existent for the masses that try isometric exercises in that manner. Hundreds of my students and friends have tried my methods, and they all receive massive growth spurts. How?
They were neglecting the density method completely at every set of their workouts.

01 DEVELOPING SELF MASTERY

So exactly how can you activate those muscle-building dormant fibers? The Iso-Bow 30 Second exercise plans are based on force production coupled with a density approach for enhancing growth factors because combining the two elements of endurance and density increases muscle growth. This takes place by extending the set you are focusing on both aspects of the endurance-oriented-2A fibers at each workout.

I've experienced fantastic gains as a result, so have many of my trainees with density specific methods. Extending time under load while combining strength and density within the workout is the best way of increasing muscle, burning fat and enhancing a lean physique.

The 30 Second Method is 100 percent more effective and is more balanced as far as building strength and muscle density is concerned. That makes it an extremely potent, muscle-enhancing protocol! An example would be to perform the chest contraction exercise, at a medium intensity and hold that contraction for 30 seconds, after that jump into another chest exercise for another 30 seconds.

All simple—and yet effective muscle-enhancing master-plan! It is a great way to get a ripped-physique ready for the summer vacation or beach time. The 30 second method works! That's because of not only force generation, but of its high density component—more contractions in less time with a strength and endurance butt kicker.

The 30 Second Method reduces body-fat at an alarming rate. It is an excellent conditioning solution, and I have used it exclusively in 2004 on every exercise for an entire 16-week pre-contest phase. The main reasons the 30 second methods works is that it allows you to reach the growth threshold without overtaxing your nervous system. Plus, without super heavy isotonic and isometric contractions that place excessive trauma on joints and connective tissues.

01 DEVELOPING SELF MASTERY

So The truth of the matter is the growth threshold. This is the point at which the level of fatigue within the muscle is high enough that a growth response is ramped. Every isotonic and isometric contraction should be to fatigue the target muscles you are contracting, which ignites and tire all the various endurance 2As to promote muscle growth and strength gains.

You need to coax the growth threshold in a timely manner. The 30 second isotonic/isometric contractions ensure that fatigue accumulates to muscle-triggering ramps. By combining various 30 second contraction exercises, the goal is to fatigue all the endurance fibers until they hit the growth threshold.

That's what the 30 Second Method is all about, achieving that critical growth threshold without overtaxing the body's recovery systems so you continue to coax ongoing, muscle growth at every workout. This generates the most force possible.

Fiber recruitment By incorporating the Iso-Bow 30 second method it places the target body-parts in an extended state, like isometric contraction/press for chest or iso-bow pull-down for lats, which is better activated with time under load. When the muscle is contracted for extended periods, the nervous system sends an emergency response signal to the brain which force muscle fibers to be recruited.

Using the 30 second method, it extends most of the fibers' attention; you use an exercise that puts the target body-part in a position to contract against resistance. This increases tension and blood blockage, and ramps up your muscle-building routine with intense muscle coaxing contractions with no relief during the set.

While performing the exercises, a tidal wave of blood rushes in, which increases a tremendous skin-stretching power-pump. For example, after a set of Iso-bow curls and Iso-concentration curls, you end your arm routine with an isometric curl for continuous muscle tension throughout the entire muscle.

01 DEVELOPING SELF MASTERY

The Tension-Overload: A 30 second blast on the targeted muscle with a certain amount of muscle-building-tension time on every exercise, increases optimal hypertrophic tension for the best muscle-stimulation to induce growth.
Most isometric books never teach trainees how to get close to the upper range of the 30 plus seconds per movement. Most usually don't even hit the minimum of 60 seconds, so that's why muscle stimulation and gains are slow for most trainees.

The 30 second method increases new muscle and strength gains. Moderate isometric contractions with a 30 second contraction allow you to continue to grow without joint stress. The 30 second method will supercharge your muscle-building results. By getting the best effects and activating most of the type 2As endurance muscle fibers. This prepares you for a new surge in muscle growth!

The Size Principle: Now let's get into the meat and potatoes of it all. The important element the trainee needs to understand to enhance and create ongoing muscle growth is the Size Principle of muscle-fiber-recruitment. The three important fiber types are: 1, 2As and 2Bs.

Type 1s These are the "supers" and are highly aerobic units, they require oxygen to fire, and they have loads of mitochondria, which is the cell's "powerhouse" and where fat is burned and used for energy. You use the type 1s when you power walk and jog.

Type 2As These fibers have both anaerobic and aerobic properties. They are used for high-intensity and low-intensity work. They have mitochondria but fewer than the type 1s.

Type 2Bs Are the "Power guys" the anaerobic power fibers—no mitochondria or oxygen required. These require low-tension time. For example, with a set of 10 reps, most of the fibers that fire first will be the 1s, followed by the 2As and, maybe some 2Bs will kick in at the very end of the set. That's the real deal with the Size Principle of fiber recruitment.

01 DEVELOPING SELF MASTERY

All fiber types will fire on the 30 second method with multi-extended sets, just in different capacities. Therefore, the resistance will be moderate and more type 1s will be activated. So heavy or strong resistance will do very little with increasing muscle size and few type 1s fire. Ultra-heavy isometric and isotonic resistance is not the best way to create ultimate muscle growth and strength gains safely. Here's why...

Using extreme or heavy isometric resistance does nothing for muscular growth, and the 2B fibers are not activated at all! Therefore, optimal isometric training for anyone interested in muscle size need to focus on the 2A power fibers, along with the endurance fibers. So once you are interested in ultimate-muscle growth, you do not have to worry about using extreme resistance. However, using extreme or very strong resistance increases strength-gains, but with the price of damaging your connective tissues in the long run.

This is where the 30 second method comes in and keeps training with isometrics safe while you build muscle and might. There is a mix of muscle and strength building while hitting those important endurance growth fibers for several reasons. To begin with, you will activate both facets of muscle expansion. With this book there is no guesswork and you exercise both the power part of the 2As (myofibrils) and the more endurance part (sarcoplasm), plus the type-1 aerobic fibers to a massive degree.

It is heavily stated by popular dogma that with isometrics training one should use strong force stating: it is the key to optimal strength gains. That's only partially true; most instructions regarding isometrics want the trainee to perform an isometric movement between 7-10 seconds max. The target muscle is only under force output for 7 seconds at most. That's only 2A power tension time that primarily affects the power fibers. You might get stronger but not bigger! By using only the 7 second time frame, loads of "endurance" muscle-building potential haven't been tapped into.

To achieve ultimate muscle growth and strength, which will be achieved with muscle-tension in the 30 second range, or tension time lasting 60-plus seconds, for 2A muscle expansion plus type-1 activation. Because of extended time under load, the 30 Second Method increases more myofibrillar thickening in the muscle, combined with isotonic exercises.

01 DEVELOPING SELF MASTERY

Everyone will build more muscle and strength, along with lean muscle size with a shredded physique, following the 30 Second Method. Performing an isometric contraction using the 30 Second Method way of training will enhance and procure an increase in **"SERIOUS MUSCLE SIZE."** Almost daily. Why is the 30 Second Method so effective?

It all begins with the size principle of fiber recruitment. My method makes it happen more thoroughly and efficiently—the extended set principal fatigues the slow-twitch fibers, but with more precision. This forces more fast-twitch-endurance-fibers to fire continuously exercise after exercise, set after set, this is exactly what you want for increasing health, strength and muscle size.

The 30 Second Method has key muscle-enhancing triggers, now with the 30 Second Method it sets the right dose which packs on lean muscle size. I have combined those with the fiber-activation supercharger to increase your strength gains through the roof.

Chapter 2:

CHEST

BUILD A POWERFUL CHEST

BUILD A POWERFUL CHEST

02 BUILD A POWERFUL CHEST

The chest muscles allow you to push or move the arm forward or across the body. These muscles are activated in any throwing or pushing motion. Aesthetically, building a powerful chest is a sign of power in men.

However, the chest muscles are not used daily, so most times they are under developed. So despite, the simplicity of how these muscles contract, they can be trained in a number of various angles of push and pull, each offer its own special muscle enhancing properties.

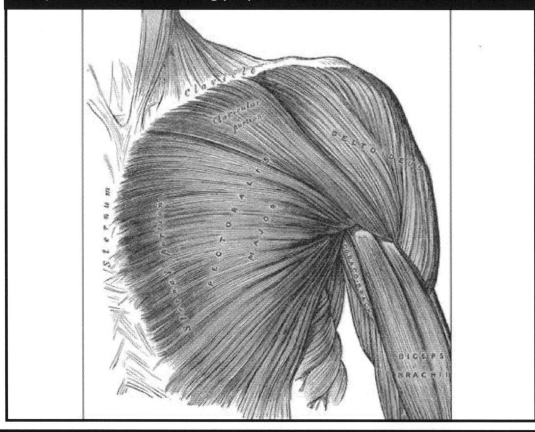

CHEST EXERCISES

02 BUILD A POWERFUL CHEST

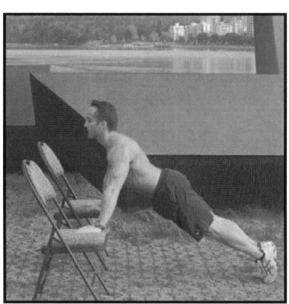

INCLINE PUSHUPS

This exercise is the Granddaddy of all upper-body exercises. It's the best upper-body builder and conditioner there is. This exercise is performed exactly as shown.

Place your hands on two chairs that are 15 inches high, the higher you go the greater pre-stretch there is. At the bottom position to enhance muscle-building stimuli, pause for 2 seconds before reversing the movement.

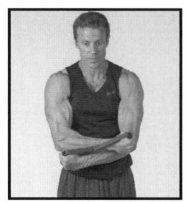
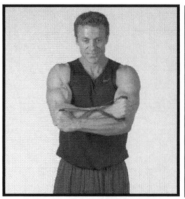
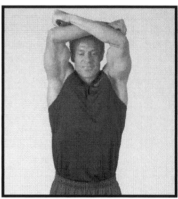

CHEST CONTRACTION

Cross arms as shown press the arms in opposite directions maintaining the tension. **(Isometric Contraction)** Now move your arm upwards and overhead, then reverse the motion maintaining strong tension. **DUAL ACTION**

Chapter 3:

SHOULDERS

DEVELOP POWERFUL SHOULDERS

DEVELOP POWERFUL SHOULDERS

03 DEVELOP POWERFUL SHOULDERS

The shoulder muscles are divided into three heads and are quite unique and move the arm in all directions. The front muscle raise the arm forward, the side muscles made up of a number of muscle bundles, and raises the arm out to the sides. The rear or posterior muscle, is designed to pull the arm backwards. Shoulder presses is a multi-muscle-use exercise, which is a compound exercise. This exercise recruits the front and side heads of the shoulders that tie in well with stimulating the upper and mid-back muscles as well giving the entire girdle complete development.

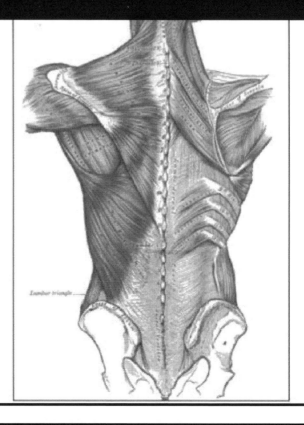

SHOULDER EXERCISES

03 DEVELOP POWERFUL SHOULDERS

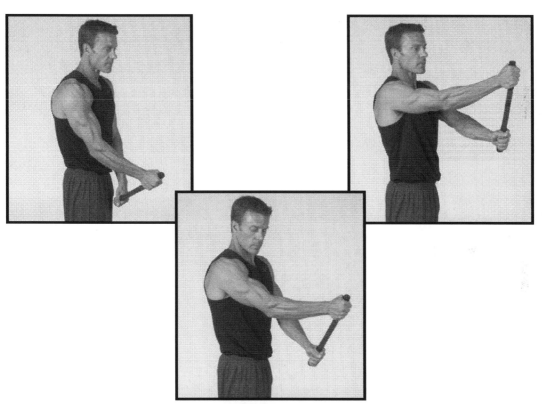

FORWARD RAISES

Grasp the Iso-Bow in front of the body, as shown. Gradually raise the arm forward against the resistance of the other hand. **RESIST IN THE UP MOTION ONLY** This works the front part of the shoulder muscles.

SHOULDER EXERCISES

03 DEVELOP BARN DOOR SHOULDERS

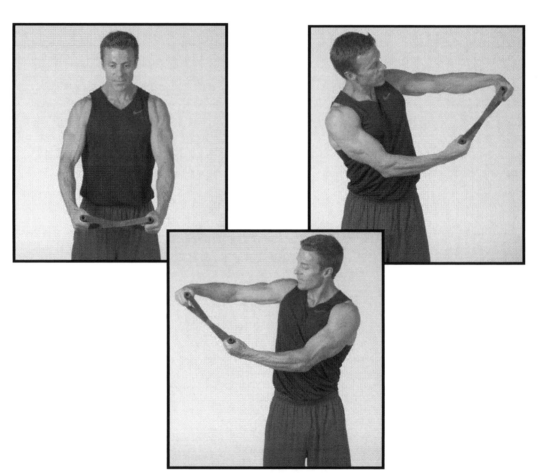

LATERAL RAISES

Hold the Iso-Bow at waist, keep your elbows slightly bent, raise your arm as shown while resisting with the other arm. Perform all reps on one side first before switching arms. **RESIST IN ONE DIRECTION ONLY**

SHOULDER EXERCISES

03 DEVELOP POWERFUL SHOULDERS

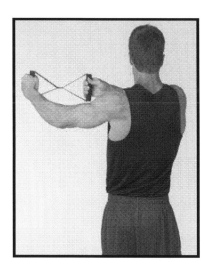 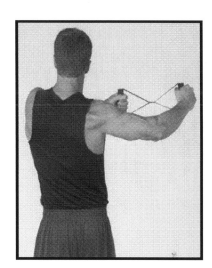

ACROSS THE BODY PULLS

Place the Iso-Bow at chest height, keep your elbows slightly bent, pull the arm toward the right while resisting with the other arm. Pause and reverse the motion alternating sides. **DUAL ACTION RESIST IN BOTH DIRECTIONS**

Chapter 4:

UPPER BACK
DEVELOP A POWERFUL V-TAPER

DEVELOP A POWERFUL V-TAPER

04 DEVELOP A POWERFUL V-TAPER

The entire back is made up of many muscles overlapping each other. However, most trainees find the back quite difficult to fully develop. The reason? As the saying goes out of sight, out of mind. We cannot directly see the back muscles, plus we cannot see it flex like we would see the biceps.

We make training the entire back musculature much easier making developing the back obviously simple once you know what you are doing, you can bring these muscles up to speed. We are looking at the large Latissimus that covers the majority of the back. The trapezius is broken up into two sections.

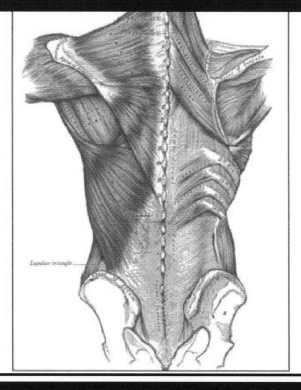

UPPER BACK EXERCISES

04 DEVELOP A POWERFUL V-TAPER

DO NOT NEGLECT THE MID AND LOWER TRAPS

The upper traps and mid-back muscles. Plus, we have the teres major, which is strongly stimulated with unilateral work, which makes self resistance the ideal movement. The infraspinatus muscle is like a half circle on each side of the upper back and is a very important rotator cuff muscle.

This muscle stabilizes the shoulder and prevents dislocations. Even though this muscle is at the back, most traditional exercises do not fully target these muscles. However, with self resistance there are exercises that target this area for full development.

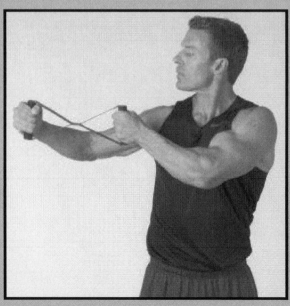

UPPER BACK EXERCISES

04 DEVELOP A POWERFUL V-TAPER

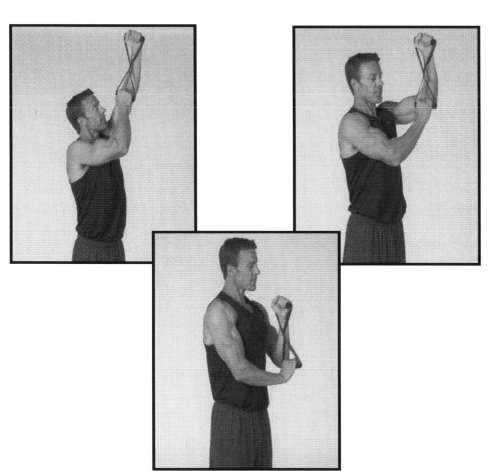

PULLDOWNS

Grasp the Iso-Bow as shown in the picture. Gradually pull the arm downwards while resisting with the bottom arm.**RESIST IN ONE DIRECTION ONLY**

UPPER BACK EXERCISES

04 DEVELOP A POWERFUL V-TAPER

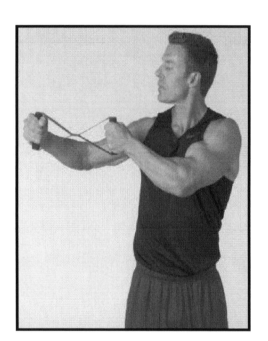 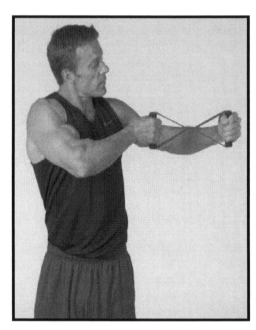

UPPER BACK ROWS

Bring your arm across the body pre-stretching the mid-back, grasp the Iso-Bow as shown. Slowly pull the arm across the body toward the armpit against the resistance supplied by the other arm. Extend the arm back to the starting position. Repeat the movement, then switch arms. This adds thickens to the mid-back, lats, and triceps along with the rear part of the shoulders.
RESIST IN A DUAL MANNER

UPPER BACK EXERCISES

04 DEVELOP A POWERFUL V-TAPER

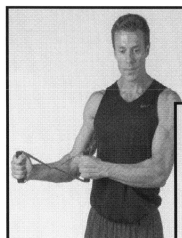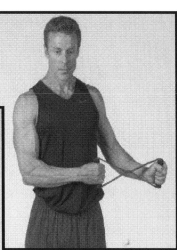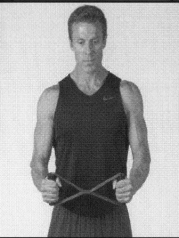

ADD POWER TO THE ROTATOR CUFF MUSCLES

Hold the Iso-Bow as shown. Pull the arms towards the middle of the exercise position, pause for 1 second, then proceed to the opposite side. **RESIST IN A DUAL MANNER**

Chapter 5:

BICEPS

DEVELOP POWERFUL BICEPS

DEVELOP POWERFUL BICEPS

05 DEVELOP POWERFUL BICEPS

The biceps muscle has two heads. A short head, which is on the inside of the arm, and a long head, which is on the outside. This is the part that people see first. The main roll of the biceps is to flex the forearm by bringing the hand towards the shoulder. In order to build powerful complete biceps, you need to learn that the biceps do not work by itself.

The brachialis, which is under the bicep when developed, gives the bicep a larger and fuller appearance. Performing curls place undesirable tension on the tendon near the elbow. In other words, the biceps is placed in a very vulnerable position. Always start all bicep exercises with a slight bend at the start and finish. Always maintain tension on the biceps and not the joint.

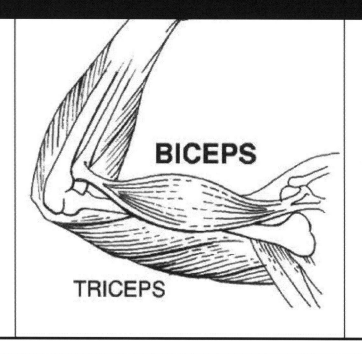

BICEPS

TRICEPS

BICEP EXERCISES

05 DEVELOP POWERFUL BICEPS

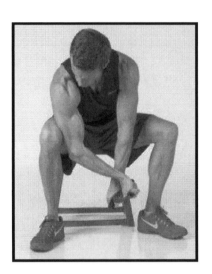 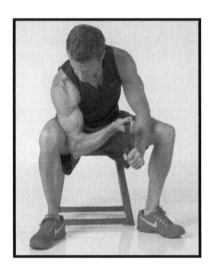

CONCENTRATION CURLS

As pictured, pull the right arm towards the face while resisting with the left hand. Now reverse the exercise by pushing the left arm down and resisting with the right. Complete your reps then switch arms and repeat movement. **DUAL ACTION**

BICEP EXERCISES

05 DEVELOP POWERFUL BICEPS

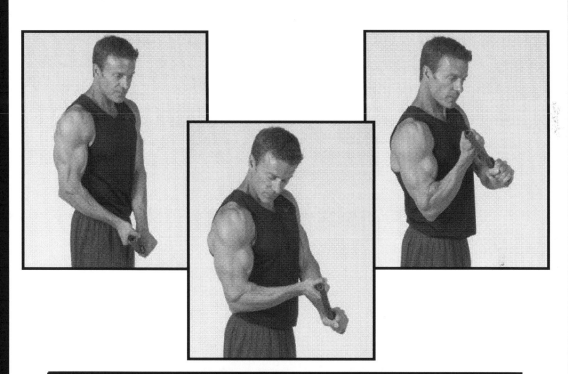

PALM UP CURLS

Pull the right arm upward towards the shoulder while resisting with the left hand. At the shoulder, reverse the exercise by pushing the left arm downwards, resisting with the right.

Chapter 6:

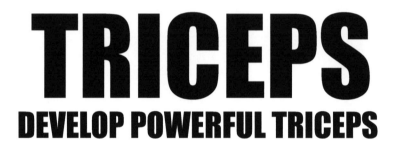

TRICEPS
DEVELOP POWERFUL TRICEPS

DEVELOP POWERFUL TRICEPS

06 DEVELOP POWERFUL TRICEPS

DEVELOP POWERFUL TRICEPS

The triceps has three heads: The lateral head, middle head and the long head. The role of the triceps is to straighten the arm. The triceps work in opposition to the biceps and brachialis muscles. The triceps has three heads this makes it much larger in mass than the biceps and the brachialis.

Unfortunately, most pay attention to the biceps, leaving the triceps underdeveloped. The lateral head, which is on the outside is what people see first. The triceps are easy to develop and we have made it easy for the trainee to achieve this.

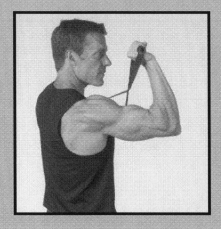

TRICEP EXERCISES

06 DEVELOP POWERFUL TRICEPS

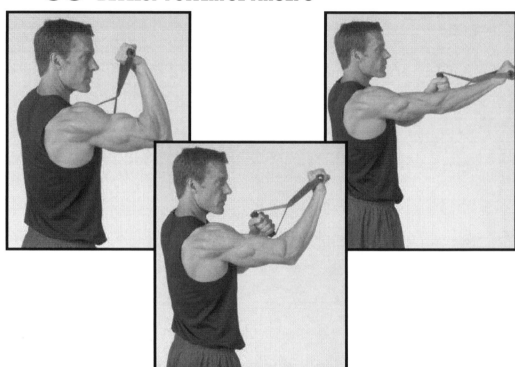

FORWARD EXTENSIONS

As shown above, press the right arm forward while resisting with the left hand. **Do not straighten the elbow.**
RESIST IN A DUAL MANNER

TRICEP EXERCISES

06 DEVELOP POWERFUL TRICEPS

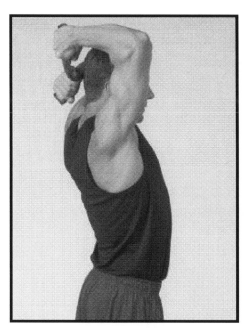 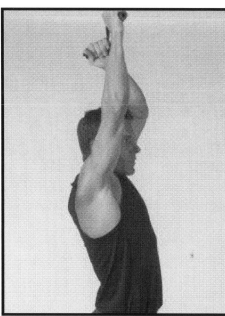

OVERHEAD TRICEP EXTENSIONS

Place arms overhead, press the right arm upwards while resisting with the left arm. Use a light to moderate tension due to the tricep tendons being sensitive at that position. **Do not straighten the elbow. RESIST IN ONE DIRECTION ONLY**

TRICEP EXERCISES

06 DEVELOP POWERFUL TRICEPS

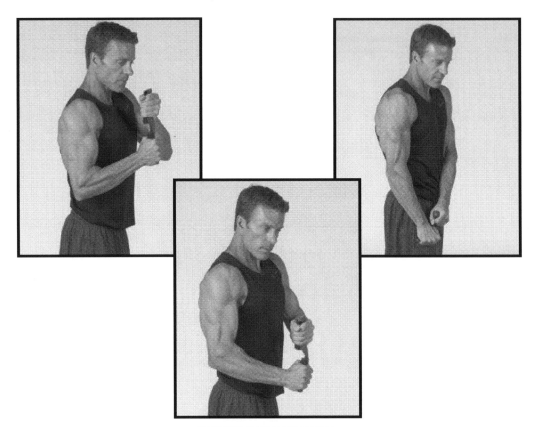

TRICEP PRESSDOWN

As pictured above, press the right hand downwards while resisting with the left arm. Repeat desired reps then switch arms. **RESIST IN ONE DIRECTION ONLY**

DEVELOP RIPPED FOREARMS

07 DEVELOP RIPPED FOREARMS

DEVELOP RIPPED FOREARMS

DEVELOP RIPPED FOREARMS

Forearm muscles are involved in every daily activity, just like the calves and abdominals. We use these muscles all the time, when we drive, write, type, hold a bag and even open a door.

Many of the muscles of the forearm deal with Muscle-multi-use. When you are moving the elbow by lowering and raising the forearm. Moving the wrist up and down by, plus raising and lowering the hand. All self resistance exercises stress the forearms to contract which will increase your grip strength.

FOREARM EXERCISES

07 DEVELOP RIPPED FOREARMS

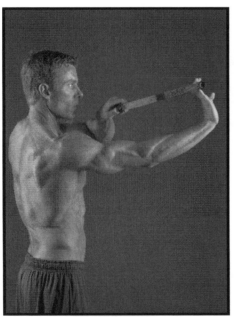
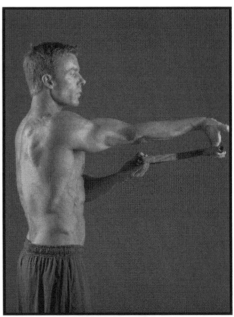

EXERCISE ONE   **EXERCISE TWO**

HAND/FOREARM EXERCISE

EXERCISE ONE: As pictured press the right hand forward until the fingers are pointed towards your feet. Return to position and repeat. **RESIST IN ONE DIRECTION**

EXERCISE TWO: Same as exercise one but, the hand is placed downwards.

Chapter 8:

THIGHS
DEVELOP POWERFUL THIGHS

DEVELOP POWERFUL TIRELESS THIGHS

08 DEVELOP POWERFUL TIRELESS THIGHS

DEVELOP POWERFUL THIGHS

The thigh muscles are basically made up of four main muscles: the vastus lateral muscle, this is located on the outside of the thighs. The vastus medial muscle, this is located on the inside of the thigh muscles towards the knee.

Better known as the tear drop because of its shape. The recus-femoris, which is located in the center of the muscles, and the vastus intermedius, this muscle is mostly covered by all the other muscles of the thighs. The Power Iso-Bow Transformation Method will develop tireless thighs with a power pack punch.

LEG EXERCISES

08 DEVELOP POWERFUL TIRELESS THIGHS

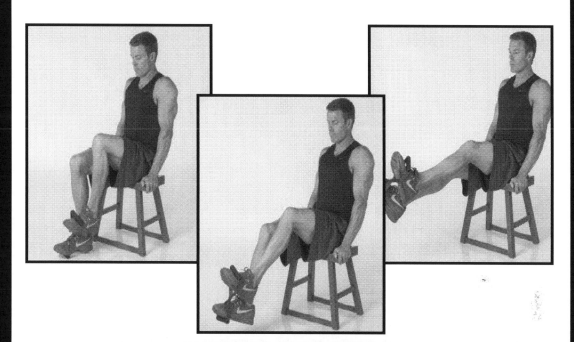

LEG EXTENSIONS

While seated on a chair, box or stool, place the legs as shown in the picture. Now extend the left leg outwards resisting with the right. At the top pause for 2 seconds, then reverse the movement by pulling down with the right while resisting with the left. **DO NOT STRAIGHTEN THE KNEE. RESIST IN A DUAL MANNER**

LEG EXERCISES

08 DEVELOP POWERFUL TIRELESS THIGHS

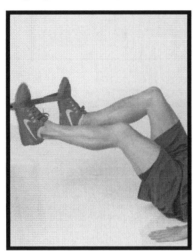 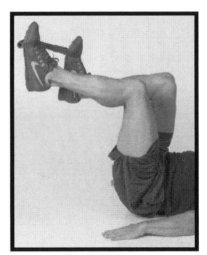

LEG PRESS

As shown, pull the right leg towards the chest, powerfully resist ing with the left leg. At the finished position, press the left foot forward resisting with the right. **PERFORM IN A DUAL MANNER**

Chapter 9:

LOWER BACK
DEVELOP POWERFUL LOWER-BACK MUSCLES

DEVELOP POWERFUL LOWER BACK MUSCLES

09 DEVELOP POWERFUL LOWER-BACK MUSCLES

POWERFUL LOWER BACK MUSCLES

Develop Powerful Lower back muscles

The lower back muscles support the lower part of the spine. When these muscles are well developed it builds a brace protecting the spine.

Apart from that the lower back muscles are responsible for bringing the body upright from a leaning forward position. Not only will the lower back be involved, but the glutes and hamstrings come into play.

LOWER BACK EXERCISES

09 DEVELOP POWERFUL LOWER BACK

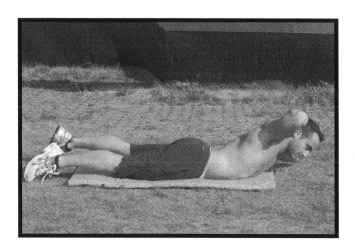

LOWER BACK EXTENSION

As shown above, this is the finished position. Lay flat on the floor and perform this movement by raising the upper body upwards slowly pause for 2 seconds at the top. Then slowly reverse the movement under control.

Chapter 10:

CALVES
DEVELOP SHAPELY CALVES

DEVELOP SHAPELY CALVES

10 DEVELOP SHAPELY CALVES

DEVELOP SHAPELY CALVES

Develop shapely calves

The calves add a finished look to the lower leg with a diamond shape. This muscle has three heads (muscle parts) the soleus, this is under the large lateral head and gives the calves a fully developed look viewed from the side and back.

The lateral and medial heads are on the outside and in the middle of the muscle. The gastrocnemius make up the majority of the calf muscle. However, the longer the gastroc, the larger the potential for enhanced calf muscle development. With The Power Iso-Bow Transformation Method the stretch component adds strength, shape and muscle development in double quick time.

DEVELOP SHAPELY CALVES

10 DEVELOP SHAPELY CALVES

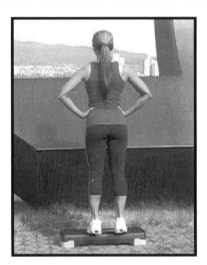 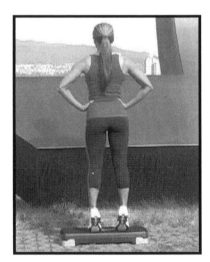

STANDING CALVE RAISES

Position yourself as shown but make sure the calves are well stretched. Start off as shown in the picture start position. Press straight up on the toes then lower. This is as awesome calve stretch exercise. Perform this exercise until the calves are well tired. This stimulates the entire calve.

Chapter 11:

ABDOMINALS
DEVELOP RIPPED ABS

DEVELOP RIPPED ABS

11 DEVELOP RIPPED ABS

The abdominal muscles are very important and reveal that the trainee has a lean physique. Plus, the role of the abdominal muscles is to protect the spine. A lean chiseled set of abdominal muscles shows the opposite sex that the owner has a sign of virility.

Once these muscles are well developed this keeps the waist line and belly flat. There are various muscle structures that complete the overall look, the entire length of the abdominal wall, plus the internal and external obliques.

The lower sections of the abdominal muscles play the largest role in protecting the spine and storing belly fat. This is the easiest place for body-fat to accumulate. Which makes training with self resistance the ideal exercise to attack those muscle fibers to the maximum.

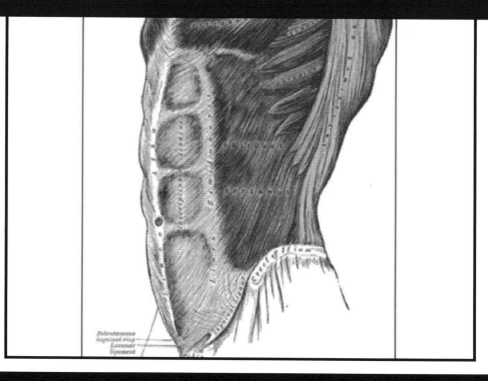

DEVELOP RIPPED ABS

11 DEVELOP RIPPED ABS

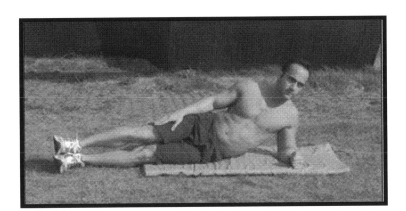

DEVELOP RIPPED ABDOMINALS

As noted in the introduction the abdominal wall includes four muscles: Let's cover the entire length from the chest to pubis is called the rectus abdominis, people say abs for short. The abdominal wall should be worked in three angles of flexion. The lower sections of the abdominal muscles. The upper sections of the abdominal wall, and the obliques. Which are rotator muscles.

DEVELOP RIPPED ABS

11 DEVELOP RIPPED ABS

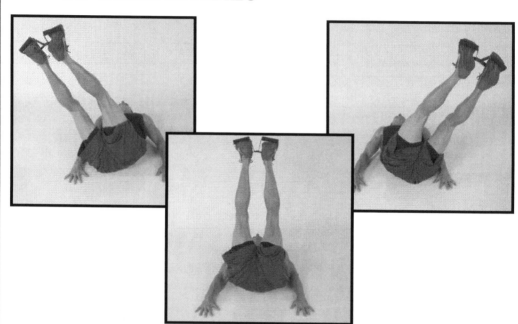

SIDE TO SIDE LATERAL RAISES

Normally people say I want to get rid of my love handles. This abdominal exercise really isolates the oblique muscles. These muscles support the spine by making the abdominal wall more rigid. Start off as shown, spread the Iso-Bow apart maintaining the tension, Then lower the legs side to side.

DEVELOP RIPPED ABS

11 DEVELOP RIPPED ABS

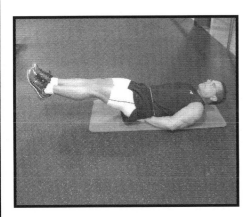 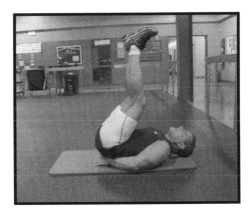

REVERSE CRUNCHES

As shown above, place your hands under your butt slowly raise the legs upwards towards the chest or stomach. Pause for a 1 second count then slowly reverse the movement. This exercise stimulates the entire abdominal wall.

DEVELOP RIPPED ABS

11 DEVELOP RIPPED ABS

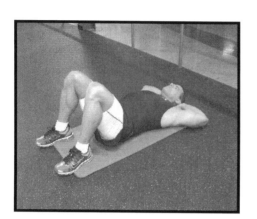 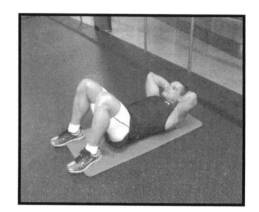

ABDOMINAL CRUNCHES

Lay on your back. Place the hands at your ear, tilt your head back, focus on the ceiling and crunch upward as shown.
DO NOT PULL ON THE HEAD.

Chapter 12:

POWER PHASE ONE METHOD

PERFORM 20 REPS, REP SPEED 2 SECONDS CONTRACTED 2 SECONDS RELEASE. ALL PHASES ARE TO BE PERFORMED FOR 2 WEEKS DO NOT SKIP PHASES

POWER PHASE METHOD PHASE ONE

12 PHASE ONE

MONDAY, WEDNESDAY, FRIDAY

Perform 2 sets of 20 reps each exercise. On the 20th rep perform a 30 second Isometric contraction. Perform each exercise using 50% of force.

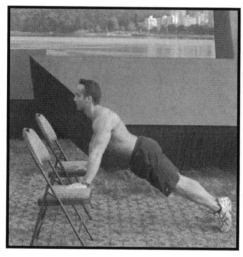
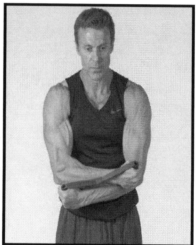

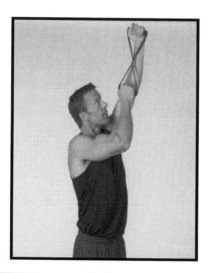
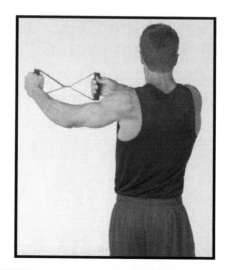

POWER PHASE METHOD PHASE ONE

12 PHASE ONE

MONDAY, WEDNESDAY, FRIDAY
Routine continued.........

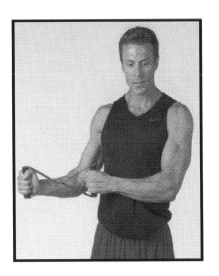

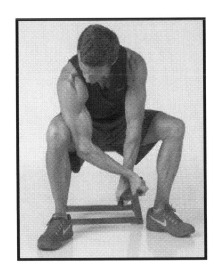

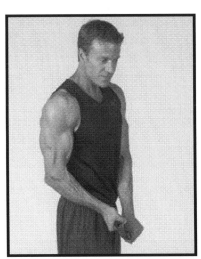

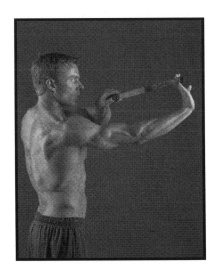

POWER PHASE METHOD PHASE ONE

12 PHASE ONE

MONDAY, WEDNESDAY, FRIDAY
Routine continued...........

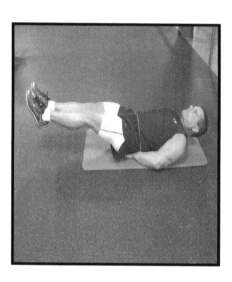 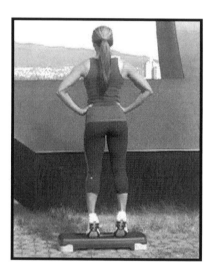

PHASE ONE MON, WED, FRI

POWER PHASE METHOD PHASE ONE

12 PHASE ONE

TUESDAY, THURSDAY, SATURDAY

Perform 2 sets of 20 reps each exercise. On the 20th rep perform a 30 second Isometric contraction. Perform each exercise using 50% of force.

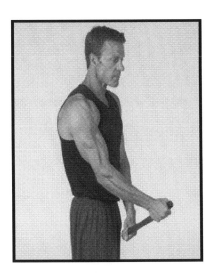
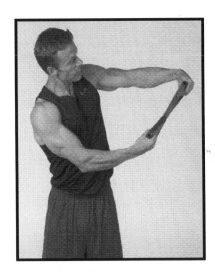
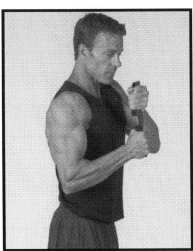
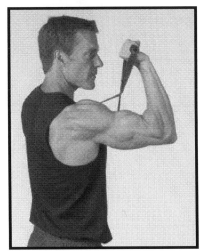

POWER PHASE METHOD PHASE ONE

12 PHASE ONE

TUESDAY, THURSDAY, SATURDAY
Continued routine..........

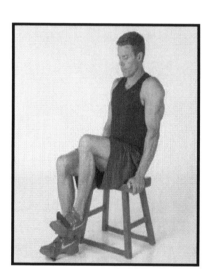
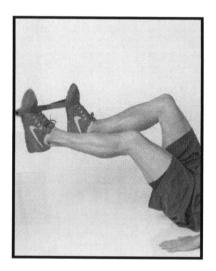

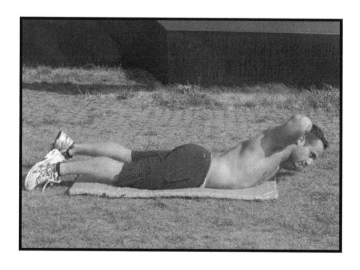

POWER PHASE METHOD PHASE ONE

12 PHASE ONE

TUESDAY, THURSDAY, SATURDAY
Continued routine........

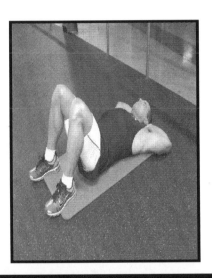 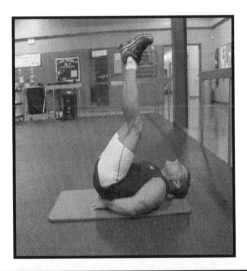

PHASE ONE TUES, THURS, SAT.

PHASE TWO

13 PHASE TWO

MONDAY, WEDNESDAY, FRIDAY

Perform 2 sets, 30 reps before moving to the next exercise. Perform each exercise using 50% of force.

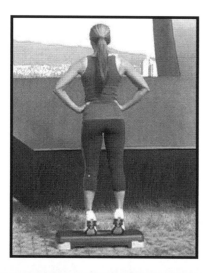
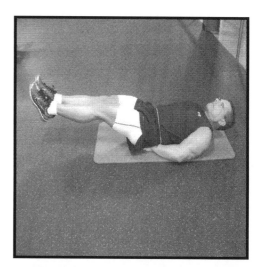
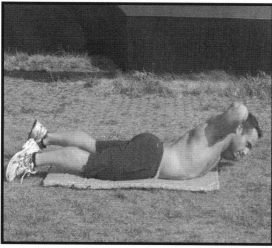
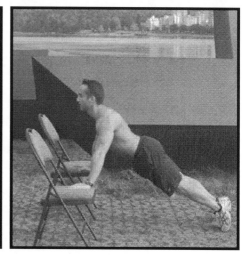

PHASE TWO

13 PHASE TWO

**MONDAY, WEDNESDAY, FRIDAY
ROUTINE CONTINUED........**

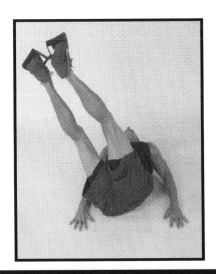
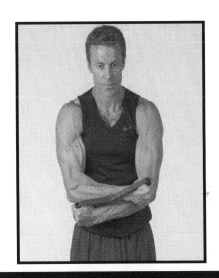

PHASE TWO   MON, WED, FRI.

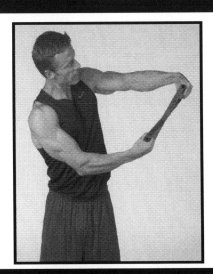
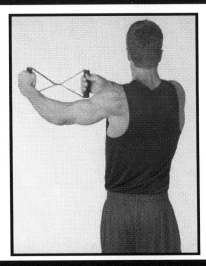

PHASE TWO

13 PHASE TWO

TUESDAY, THURSDAY, SATURDAY

Perform 30 reps at 2 sets each before moving onto the next exercise.
Perform each exercise using 50% of force.

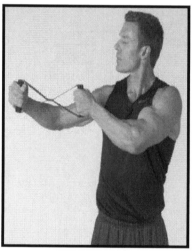
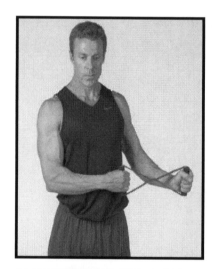
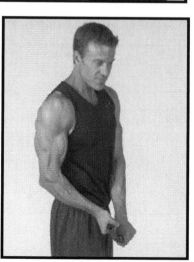
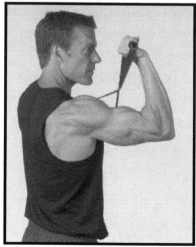

PHASE TWO

13 PHASE TWO

TUESDAY, THURSDAY, SATURDAY

ROUTINE CONTINUED..........

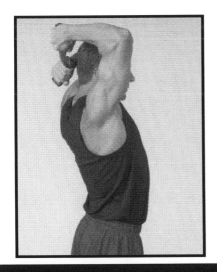
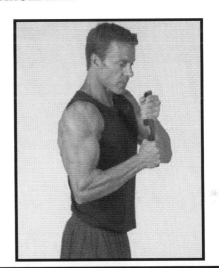

PHASE TWO   TUES, THURS, SAT.

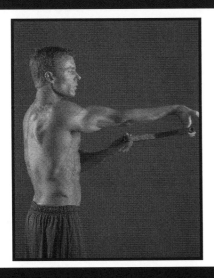
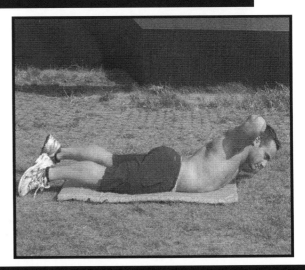

Chapter 14:

FIBER PUMP
30 PLUS

FIBER PUMP 30 PLUS METHOD
REP SPEED 2 SECOND CONTRACTION,
2 SECONDS RELEASE
2 WEEKS

30 PLUS METHOD

14 30 PLUS METHOD

HOW TO PERFORM THIS ROUTINE:
Perform 2 sets before moving to the next exercise. On the 30th rep perform a 10 second Isometric contraction at the middle section of the exercise stroke. Perform one set each exercise using 50% of force.

DAY ONE

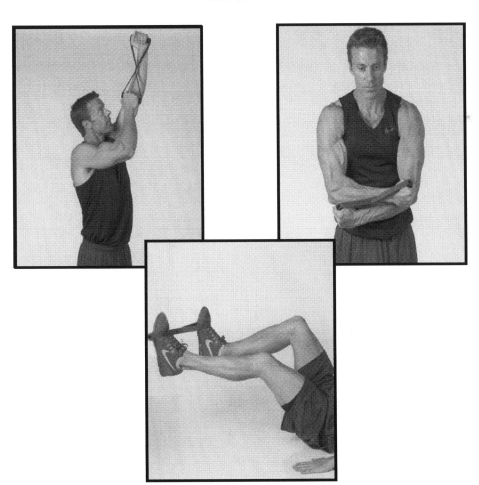

30 PLUS METHOD

14 30 PLUS METHOD

HOW TO PERFORM THIS ROUTINE:

Perform 2 sets before moving to the next exercise. On the 30th rep perform a 10 second Isometric contraction at the middle section of the exercise stroke. Perform one set each exercise using 50% of force.

DAY ONE continued.........

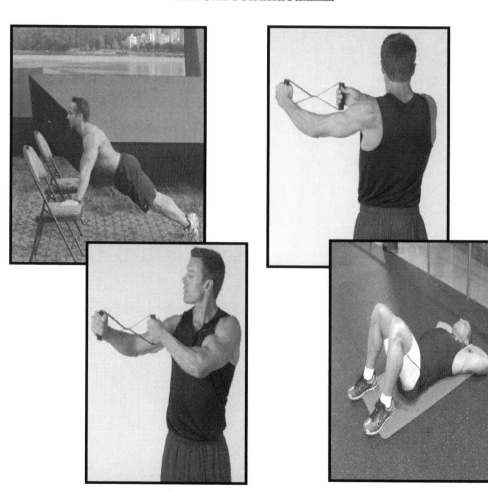

30 PLUS METHOD

14 30 PLUS METHOD

HOW TO PERFORM THIS ROUTINE:

Perform 2 sets before moving to the next exercise. On the 30th rep perform a 10 second Isometric contraction at the middle section of the exercise stroke. Perform one set each exercise using 50% of force.

DAY TWO

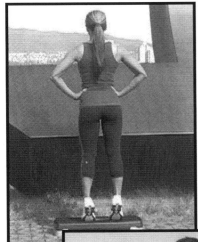
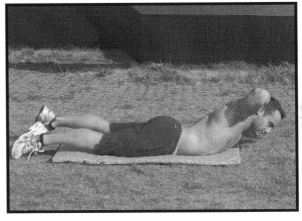
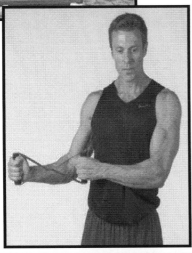
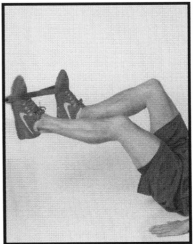

30 PLUS METHOD

14 30 PLUS METHOD

HOW TO PERFORM THIS ROUTINE:
Perform 2 sets before moving to the next exercise. On the 30th rep perform a 10 second Isometric contraction at the middle section of the exercise stroke. Perform one set each exercise using 50% of force.

DAY TWO continued.............

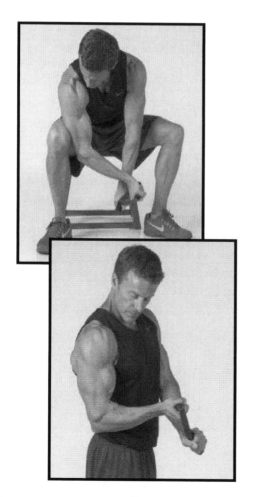
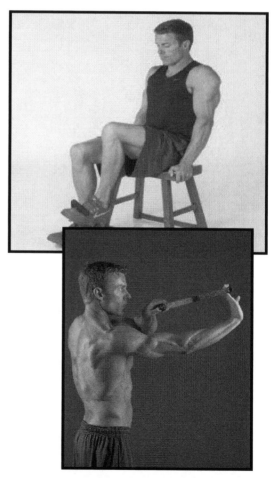

30 PLUS METHOD

14 30 PLUS METHOD

HOW TO PERFORM THIS ROUTINE:

Perform 2 sets before moving to the next exercise. On the 30th rep perform a 10 second Isometric contraction at the middle section of the exercise stroke. Perform one set each exercise using 50% of force.

DAY THREE

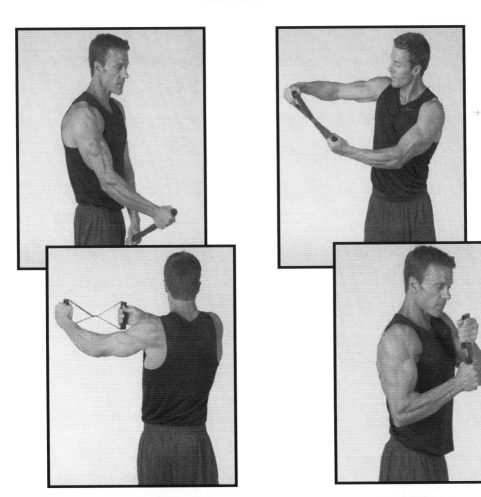

30 PLUS METHOD

14 30 PLUS METHOD

HOW TO PERFORM THIS ROUTINE:

Perform 2 sets before moving to the next exercise. On the 30th rep perform a 10 second Isometric contraction at the middle section of the exercise stroke. Perform one set each exercise using 50% of force.

DAY THREE continued.......

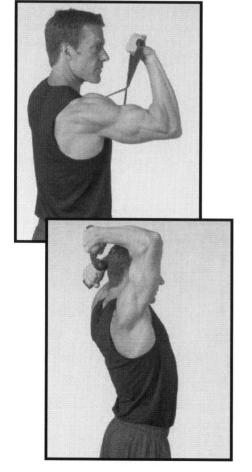
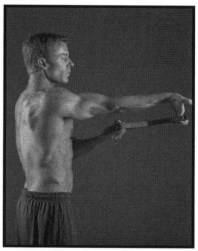
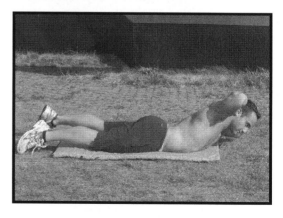

30 PLUS METHOD

14 30 PLUS METHOD

HOW TO PERFORM THIS ROUTINE:

Perform 2 sets before moving to the next exercise. On the 30th rep perform a 10 second Isometric contraction at the middle section of the exercise stroke. Perform one set each exercise using 50% of force.

DAY THREE continued.......

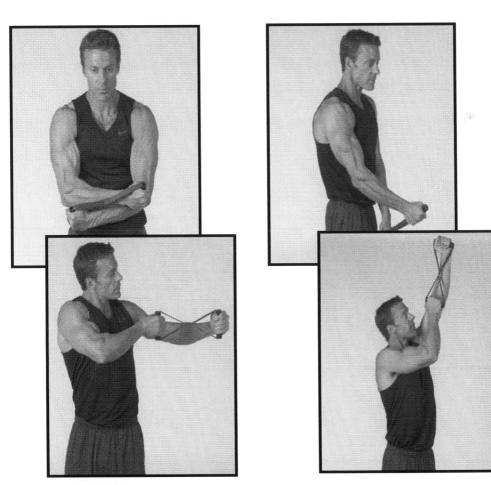

30 PLUS METHOD

14 30 PLUS METHOD

HOW TO PERFORM THIS ROUTINE:

Perform 2 sets before moving to the next exercise. On the 30th rep perform a 10 second Isometric contraction at the middle section of the exercise stroke. Perform one set each exercise using 50% of force.

DAY FOUR

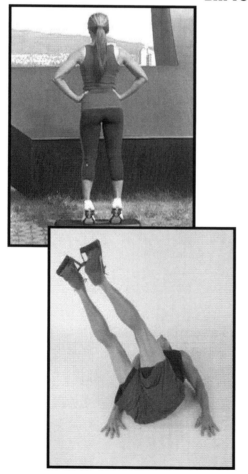
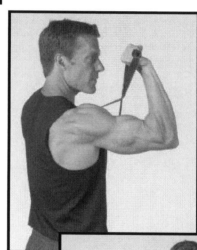
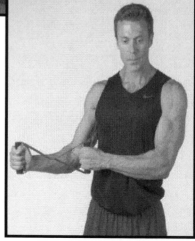

30 PLUS METHOD

14 30 PLUS METHOD

HOW TO PERFORM THIS ROUTINE:

Perform 2 sets before moving to the next exercise. On the 30th rep perform a 10 second Isometric contraction at the middle section of the exercise stroke. Perform one set each exercise using 50% of force.

DAY FOUR continued......

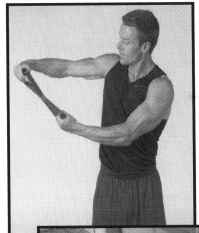

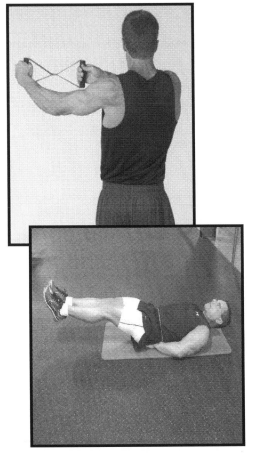

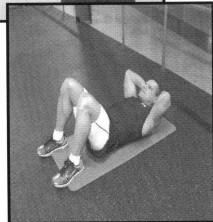

30 PLUS METHOD

14 30 PLUS METHOD

HOW TO PERFORM THIS ROUTINE:

Perform 2 sets before moving to the next exercise. On the 30th rep perform a 10 second Isometric contraction at the middle section of the exercise stroke. Perform one set each exercise using 50% of force.

DAY FIVE

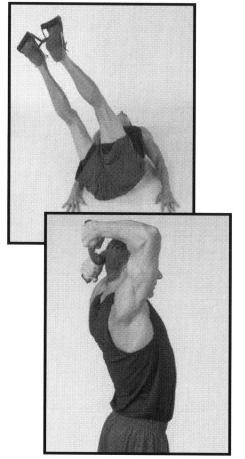
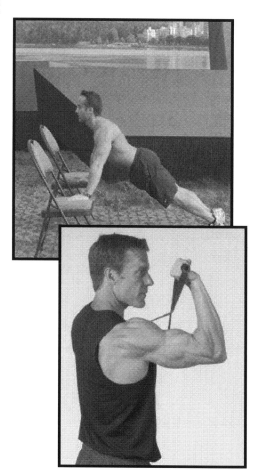

30 PLUS METHOD

14 30 PLUS METHOD

HOW TO PERFORM THIS ROUTINE:

Perform 2 sets before moving to the next exercise. On the 30th rep perform a 10 second Isometric contraction at the middle section of the exercise stroke. Perform one set each exercise using 50% of force.

DAY FIVE continued.....

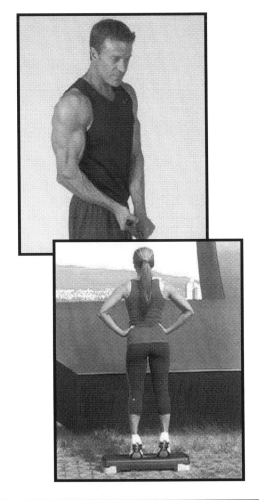

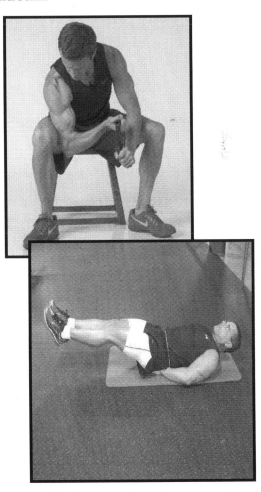

Chapter 15:

THE POWER 30 HYPER-GROWTH PROGRAM PHASE ONE

THE POWER 30 HYPER-GROWTH PROGRAM

15 THE POWER 30 HYPER-GROWTH PROGRAM

HOW TO PERFORM THIS ROUTINE:
PHASE ONE HYPER PHASE

Perform 30 reps, followed by a 30 second isometric contraction at the contracted position. One set per exercise. **REP SPEED 2 SECONDS CONTRACTED, 2 SECONDS RELEASE**

DAY ONE

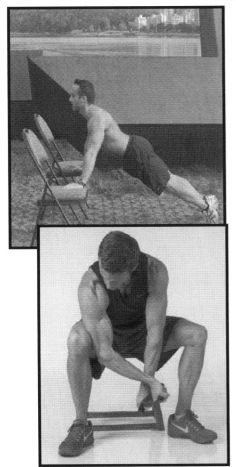

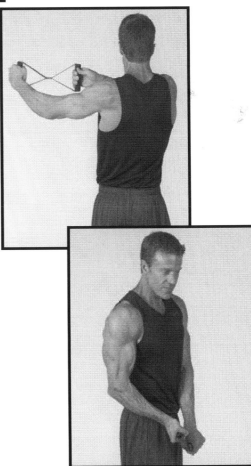

THE POWER 30 HYPER-GROWTH PROGRAM

15 THE POWER 30 HYPER-GROWTH PROGRAM

HOW TO PERFORM THIS ROUTINE:
PHASE ONE HYPER PHASE

Perform 30 reps, followed by a 30 second isometric contraction at the contracted position. One set per exercise. **REP SPEED 2 SECONDS CONTRACTED, 2 SECONDS RELEASE**

DAY ONE continued............

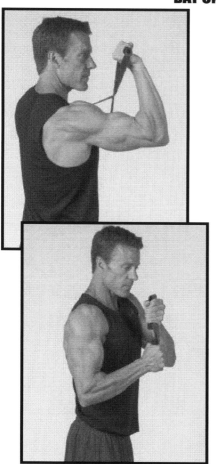

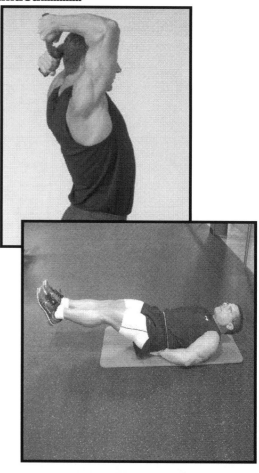

THE POWER 30 HYPER-GROWTH PROGRAM

15 THE POWER 30 HYPER-GROWTH PROGRAM

HOW TO PERFORM THIS ROUTINE:
PHASE ONE HYPER PHASE

Perform 30 reps, followed by a 30 second isometric contraction at the contracted position. One set per exercise. **REP SPEED 2 SECONDS CONTRACTED, 2 SECONDS RELEASE**

DAY TWO

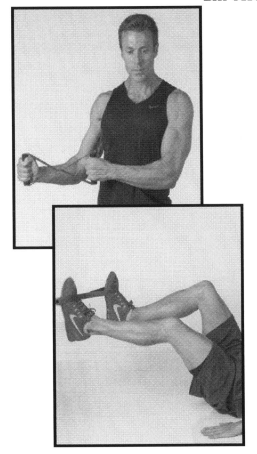
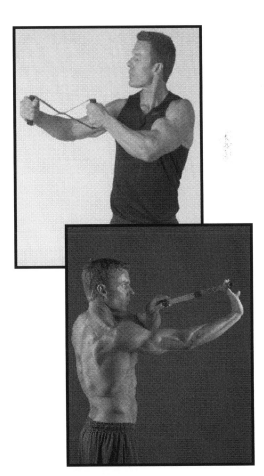

THE POWER 30 HYPER-GROWTH PROGRAM

15 THE POWER 30 HYPER-GROWTH PROGRAM

HOW TO PERFORM THIS ROUTINE:
PHASE ONE HYPER PHASE

Perform 30 reps, followed by a 30 second isometric contraction at the contracted position. One set per exercise. **REP SPEED 2 SECONDS CONTRACTED, 2 SECONDS RELEASE**

DAY TWO continued.......

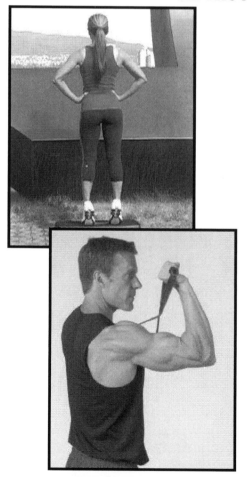

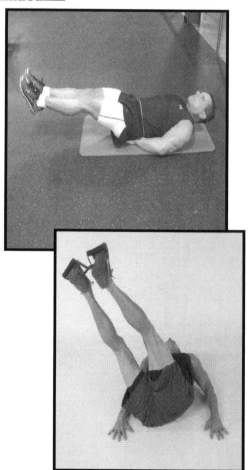

THE POWER 30 HYPER-GROWTH PROGRAM

15 THE POWER 30 HYPER-GROWTH PROGRAM

HOW TO PERFORM THIS ROUTINE:
PHASE ONE HYPER PHASE

Perform 30 reps, followed by a 30 second isometric contraction at the contracted position. One set per exercise. **REP SPEED 2 SECONDS CONTRACTED, 2 SECONDS RELEASE**

DAY THREE

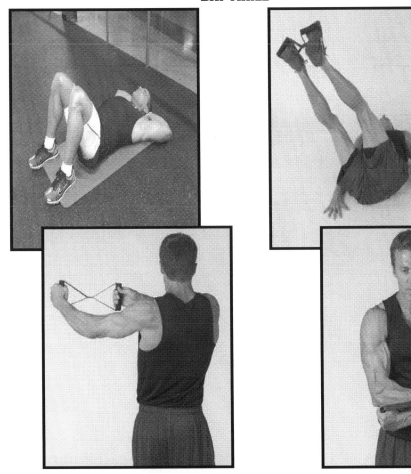

THE POWER 30 HYPER-GROWTH PROGRAM

15 THE POWER 30 HYPER-GROWTH PROGRAM

HOW TO PERFORM THIS ROUTINE:
PHASE ONE HYPER PHASE

Perform 30 reps, followed by a 30 second isometric contraction at the contracted position. One set per exercise. **REP SPEED 2 SECONDS CONTRACTED, 2 SECONDS RELEASE**

DAY THREE continued..........

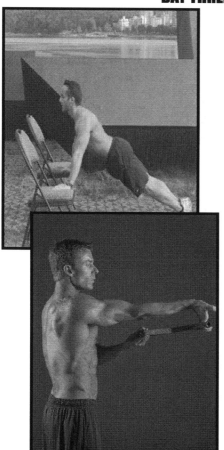

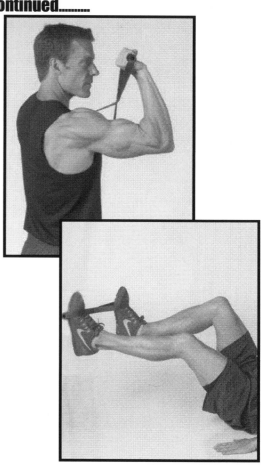

THE POWER 30 HYPER-GROWTH PROGRAM

15 THE POWER 30 HYPER-GROWTH PROGRAM

HOW TO PERFORM THIS ROUTINE:
PHASE ONE HYPER PHASE

Perform 30 reps, followed by a 30 second isometric contraction at the contracted position. One set per exercise. **REP SPEED 2 SECONDS CONTRACTED, 2 SECONDS RELEASE**

DAY FOUR

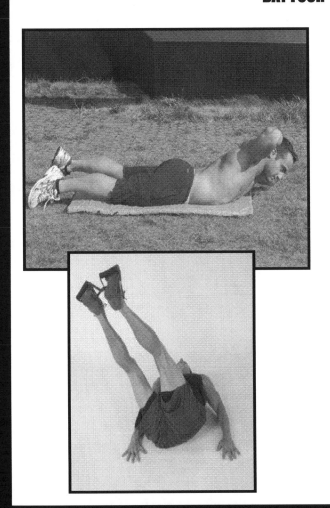

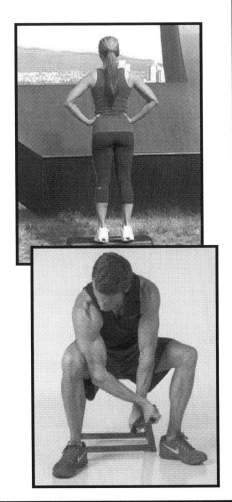

THE POWER 30 HYPER-GROWTH PROGRAM

15 THE POWER 30 HYPER-GROWTH PROGRAM

HOW TO PERFORM THIS ROUTINE:
PHASE ONE HYPER PHASE

Perform 30 reps, followed by a 30 second isometric contraction at the contracted position. One set per exercise. **REP SPEED 2 SECONDS CONTRACTED, 2 SECONDS RELEASE**

DAY FIVE

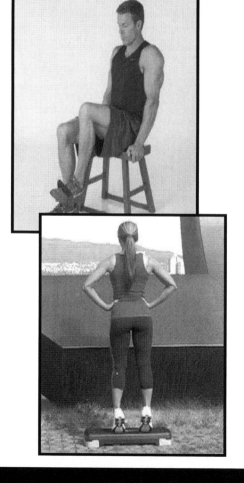

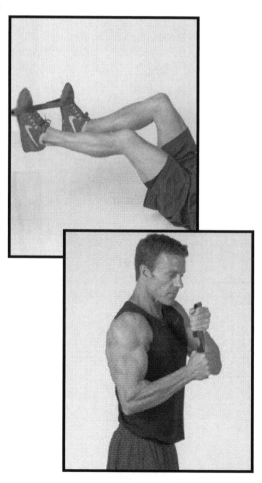

THE POWER 30 HYPER-GROWTH PROGRAM

15 THE POWER 30 HYPER-GROWTH PROGRAM

HOW TO PERFORM THIS ROUTINE:
PHASE ONE HYPER PHASE

Perform 30 reps, followed by a 30 second isometric contraction at the contracted position. One set per exercise. **REP SPEED 2 SECONDS CONTRACTED, 2 SECONDS RELEASE**

DAY FIVE continued............

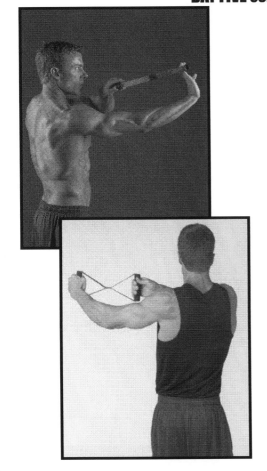
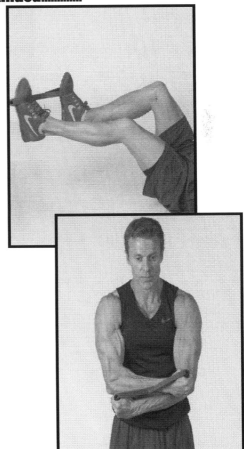

Chapter 15:

THE POWER 30 HYPER GROWTH PROGRAM PHASE TWO

THE POWER 30 HYPER-GROWTH PROGRAM

15 THE POWER 30 HYPER-GROWTH PROGRAM

HOW TO PERFORM THIS ROUTINE:
PHASE TWO

Contract within 2 seconds then slowly reverse the movement for 6 seconds. Perform 5 reps. On the 5th perform an isometric hold for 30 seconds. Alternate day one and day two for 6 days per week. One set per exercise. Perform this program for 2 weeks.

DAY ONE

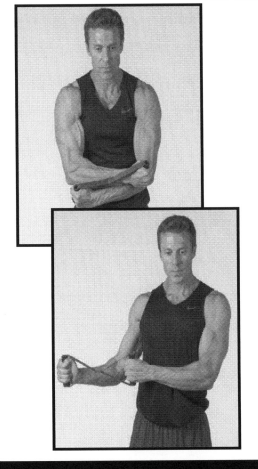

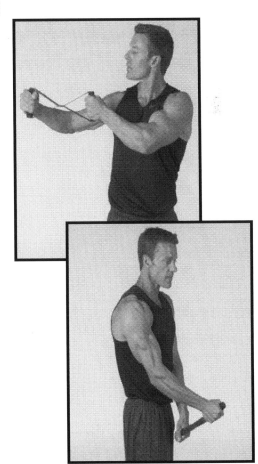

THE POWER 30 HYPER-GROWTH PROGRAM

15 THE POWER 30 HYPER-GROWTH PROGRAM

HOW TO PERFORM THIS ROUTINE:
PHASE TWO

Contract within 2 seconds then slowly reverse the movement for 6 seconds. Perform 5 reps. On the 5th perform an isometric hold for 30 seconds. Alternate day one and day two for 6 days per week. One set per exercise. Perform this program for 2 weeks.

DAY ONE continued..........

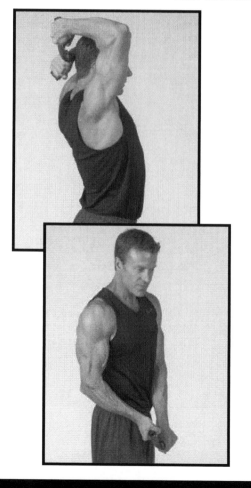

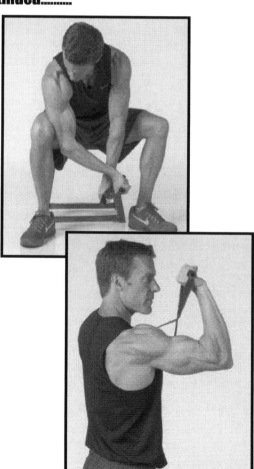

THE POWER 30 HYPER-GROWTH PROGRAM

15 THE POWER 30 HYPER-GROWTH PROGRAM

HOW TO PERFORM THIS ROUTINE:
PHASE TWO

Contract within 2 seconds then slowly reverse the movement for 6 seconds. Perform 5 reps. On the 5th perform an isometric hold for 30 seconds. Alternate day one and day two for 6 days per week. One set per exercise. Perform this program for 2 weeks.

DAY TWO

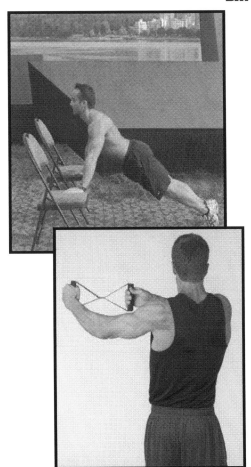

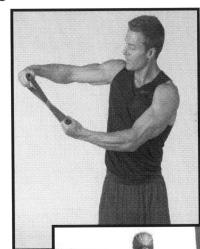

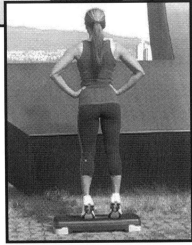

THE POWER 30 HYPER-GROWTH PROGRAM

15 THE POWER 30 HYPER-GROWTH PROGRAM

HOW TO PERFORM THIS ROUTINE:
PHASE TWO

Contract within 2 seconds then slowly reverse the movement for 6 seconds. Perform 5 reps. On the 5th perform an isometric hold for 30 seconds. Alternate day one and day two for 6 days per week. One set per exercise. Perform this program for 2 weeks.

DAY TWO continued........

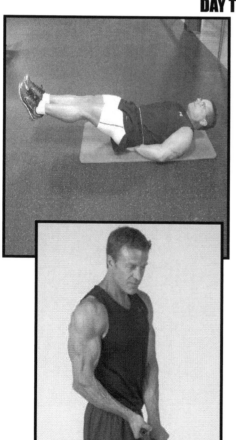

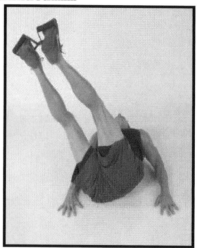

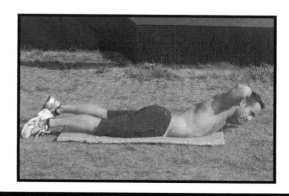

Chapter 15:

THE POWER 30 HYPER GROWTH PROGRAM PHASE THREE

THE POWER 30 HYPER-GROWTH PROGRAM

15 THE POWER 30 HYPER-GROWTH PROGRAM

HOW TO PERFORM THIS ROUTINE:
PHASE THREE

Perform a 30 second isometric rep then perform 30 reps —by contracting for 2 seconds and release 2 seconds. Alternate day one and day two for 6 days per week. One set each exercise.

DAY ONE

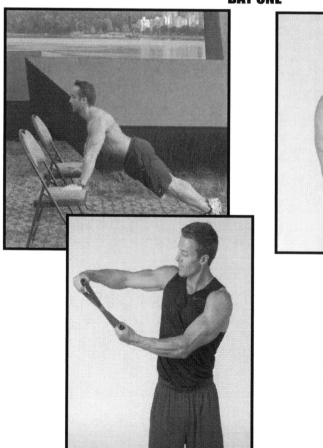

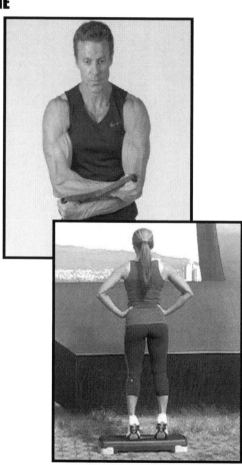

THE POWER 30 HYPER-GROWTH PROGRAM

15 THE POWER 30 HYPER-GROWTH PROGRAM

HOW TO PERFORM THIS ROUTINE:
PHASE THREE

Perform a 30 second isometric rep then perform 30 reps —by contracting for 2 seconds and release 2 seconds. Alternate day one and day two for 6 days per week. One set each exercise.

DAY ONE continued...........

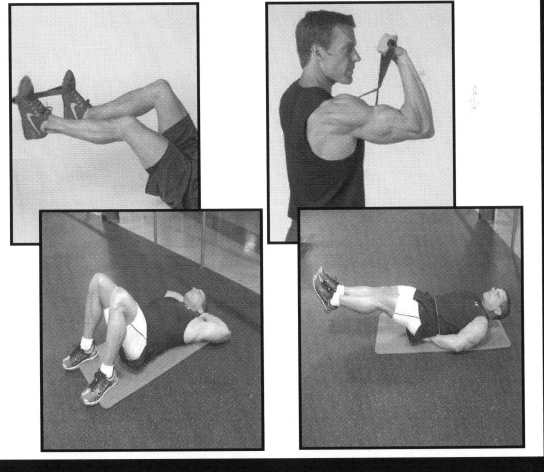

THE POWER 30 HYPER-GROWTH PROGRAM

15 THE POWER 30 HYPER-GROWTH PROGRAM

HOW TO PERFORM THIS ROUTINE:
PHASE THREE

Perform a 30 second isometric rep then perform 30 reps —by contracting for 2 seconds and release 2 seconds. Alternate day one and day two for 6 days per week. One set each exercise.

DAY TWO

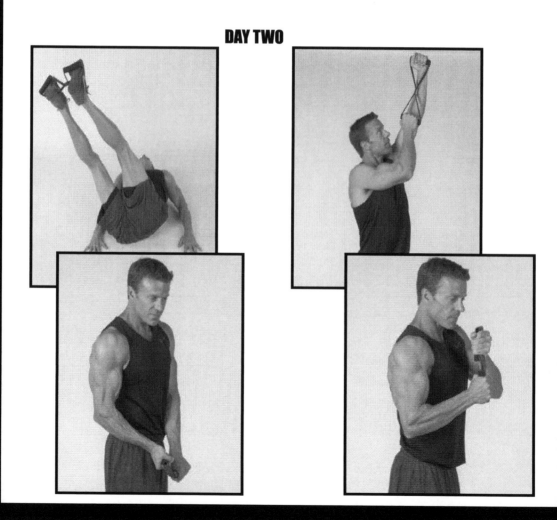

THE POWER 30 HYPER-GROWTH PROGRAM

15 THE POWER 30 HYPER-GROWTH PROGRAM

HOW TO PERFORM THIS ROUTINE:
PHASE THREE

Perform a 30 second isometric rep then perform 30 reps —by contracting for 2 seconds and release 2 seconds. Alternate day one and day two for 6 days per week. One set each exercise.

DAY TWO continued...........

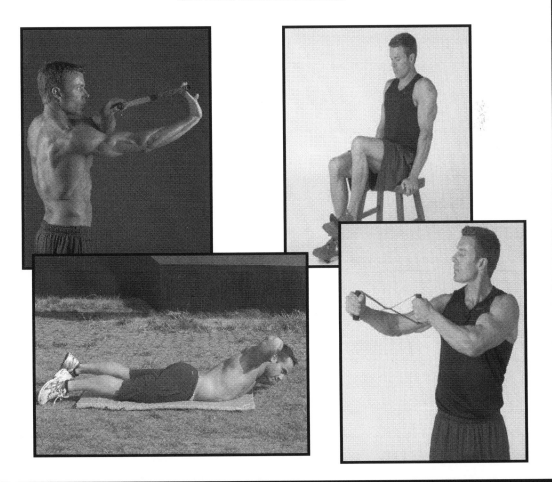

We are looking forward to hearing from you on your progress. Please drop us an email skippymarl@icloud. com

Printed in Great Britain
by Amazon

61324373R00061